Vitamins and Supplements Explained

A Look at the Vitamins and Supplements to Improve Your Health and Boost Your Immune System

Ernest Staybrook

Please consult a licensed professional before attempting any techniques outlined in this book.

By reading this document, the reader agrees that under no circumstances is the author responsible for any losses, direct or indirect, that are incurred as a result of the use of the information contained within this document, including, but not limited to, errors, omissions, or inaccuracies.

Table of Contents

Introduction

We all know vitamins are important for our health, but what do they actually do? What are the most important vitamins, and in what foods can they be found? Let's start at the basics: vitamins are organic compounds that humans need in small quantities. Vitamins are also essential nutrients we obtain from different foods. While food is a valuable source of most vitamins, there are some exceptions. Vitamin D, for instance, is not available in large enough quantities in food. Consequently, humans get the majority of their vitamin D from sunlight as the human body is able to synthesize the vitamin when exposed to it. Vitamins are incredibly important, as having a deficit of vitamins in the body can lead to health issues (Brazier, 2020).

Scientists currently recognize thirteen vitamins. These can be categorized into fat-soluble and water-soluble vitamins. One of the main differences between the two is that the former can be stored in the body for extended periods while the latter cannot. Due to this, the body needs a more frequent supply of water soluble vitamins than fat soluble ones. In this guide to vitamins, we will be exploring two fat-soluble (A and D) and two water-soluble (B and C) vitamins, as well as two important minerals (Iron and Zinc) (Brazier, 2020). We will be taking a journey through some of the most important vitamins and minerals and their health-affirming properties. Ultimately, this guide will equip you with the knowledge that, when applied, will put you on the road to becoming a fitter, healthier you.

Chapter 1: Vitamin A

Vitamin A is a fat-soluble nutrient that is important for our vision, growth, reproduction, and immune system (Mayo Clinic Staff, 2020). In the case of the latter, vitamin A plays an important role in ensuring our body's immune system can form a natural defense against illness and infection. Naturally, this makes it very important. Vitamin A also assists in day-to-day bodily functions such as improving our vision in dim light and keeping our skin healthy (NHS Choices, 2019). Vitamin A is integral to eyesight as it is an essential part of the protein rhodopsin which absorbs light in the eye receptors (National Institutes of Health, 2017).

Vitamin A deficiency is relatively low in developed countries. However, in developing countries, a vitamin A deficiency is more common and often poses serious health risks for infants and young children. These children with vitamin A deficiencies run the risk of developing blindness as well as anemia and measles (National Institutes of Health, 2017).

Where Can I Find Vitamin A?

Now that you know the perks, you've got to be wondering where you can find these essential nutrients. Luckily, a balanced diet will usually offer you all the vitamin A you need. It is also found in a variety of different foods, giving you many options to choose from. These foods include dairy products, liver, and carrots. Green vegetables such as spinach are also a fine source of vitamin A. Vitamin A also has antioxidant properties; this means that it protects the cells against free radicals, harmful molecules produced when the body is exposed to tobacco smoke or radiation. Alternatively, there is the option of taking vitamin A supplements. These can be of huge benefit to those with a limited diet or people with a condition such as pancreatic disease, increasing the body's demand for vitamin A (Mayo Clinic Staff, 2020). Chapter 2:

Vitamin B

Vitamin B refers to a class of eight different B vitamins that assist a variety of enzymes in their functions. These functions include releasing energy from carbohydrates and fat, breaking down amino acids, and transporting oxygen around the body. These eight B vitamins are: B1 (thiamin), B2 (Riboflavin), B3 (niacin), B5 (pantothenic acid), B6 (pyridoxine), B7 (biotin), B9 (folic acid), B12 (cobalamin) (*B Vitamins*, 2019). These vitamins are grouped together as they are generally found in the same foods. Each B vitamin actually has its own unique function and is needed in different amounts. For example, vitamin B2 is responsible for energy release and helps the body to absorb nutrients, while vitamin B9 is essential during pregnancy to prevent neural tube defects in babies. In terms of the recommended dose, men and women require between 1.1 and 1.3mg of B2 per day while pregnant women require 400mcg of B9 per day until they are 12 weeks pregnant (*What does Vitamin B Do? | Foods & Sources | Holland & Barrett*, n.d.).

Symptoms of a vitamin B deficiency can be quite serious, ranging from fatigue, diarrhea, and nausea. Approximately 75% of women do not get enough B9 during pregnancy which has the potential to negatively impact fetal health. B12 deficiencies are most common in vegans and the elderly as vegans eat a mostly plant-based diet. The elderly produce too little 'intrinsic factor' in their stomach; this is a natural chemical that boosts B12 absorption (*What does Vitamin B Do? | Foods & Sources | Holland & Barrett*, n.d.).

Where Can I Find Vitamin B?

For foods rich in vitamin B, there is also a wide range of options available. Salmon is a nutritious food particularly high in vitamin B. It is high in several of the different B vitamins, including B1, B2, B3, B5, B6, and B12. Leafy green vegetables stand out for their B9 content. Raw spinach and lettuce are examples of foods that are very rich in vitamin B (*15 Healthy Foods High in B Vitamins*, 2018). Garlic is an unexpected source of vitamin B; it is, in fact, a fantastic source of vitamin B6 (*Does garlic have vitamin B?*, n.d.). Garlic also has anticoagulant properties. An anticoagulant is defined as a medicine that can prevent blood clotting. According to the University of Maryland Medical Center, garlic is recommended to help prevent blood clotting and heart disease (*Healthfully*, n.d.).

Chapter 3: Vitamin C

Long associated with boosting the human immune system, vitamin C is one of the safest and most effective nutrients. Its benefits include protection against immune system deficiencies, cardiovascular diseases, eye disease, and even skin wrinkling. Researcher Mark Moyad from the University of Michigan has boasted on its behalf, claiming that "Vitamin C has received a great deal of attention, and with good reason. Higher blood levels of vitamin C may be the ideal nutrition marker for our overall health." (M, 2008)

Vitamin C is a water-soluble vitamin that the body is unable to store or produce by itself. As a result, any excess vitamin C is excreted from the body via urine. It is generally absorbed from the food we eat. This absorption takes place in the small bowel. There is a popular belief that vitamin C can prevent the common cold. This has insufficient conclusive evidence to support this. Make no mistake, though, vitamin C is immensely valuable to the body, assisting with the body's growth and repair and playing a key role in our human systems. There is even evidence that suggests that vitamin C may play a role in the body's ability to combat certain types of cancer-causing particles (*What is vitamin C?*, n.d.).

Where Can I Find Vitamin C?

Like vitamins A and B, sufficient vitamin C can usually be found in a balanced diet. Vitamin C-rich foods include oranges, kiwis, broccoli, grapefruits, brussels sprouts, cooked cabbage, and cantaloupe. The National Institutes of Health recommend that men and women get 90 mg and 75 mg per day, respectively. A single 9-ounce glass of orange juice contains 120 mg of vitamin C (Lehman, 2015). This means it only takes one serving of orange juice a day to get your recommended daily dose! Bet you didn't think it was that easy? However, sometimes it can be difficult to find time to ensure you're getting all your vitamin C daily requirements in the busy world. That is where vitamin C supplements can come in handy. Supplements can be a quick and easy way to fit your vitamin quota. Furthermore, pineapple is another good source of vitamin C (*Vitamin C: The Healing Power Of The Pineapple*, n.d.) that possesses anticoagulant properties (ePainAssist, 2018). An added bonus to your overall health!

Chapter 4: Vitamin D

Vitamin D is another incredibly important and widely known vitamin. It is commonly associated with the sun as sunlight allows the human body to synthesize it for further use. However, you'd be forgiven for not knowing exactly what it does. Vitamin D is a fat-soluble vitamin that helps with calcium absorption. Without enough vitamin D, it is impossible for the body to absorb all of the calcium it needs. Calcium famously improves bone health, and therefore vitamin D is integral to keeping our bones healthy and strong. Like other essential vitamins, vitamin D also assists with cell growth and boosts our immune system (*Vitamins & Minerals: What is Vitamin D?*, n.d.).

Unlike other vitamins A or B, vitamin D deficiency is more common as many people do not get enough sunlight to produce adequate vitamin D. When vitamin D is in short supply, children in particular, run the risk of developing rickets, a condition that causes bones to bend and weaken. Adults who have a vitamin D deficiency have another potential condition to contend with: osteoporosis. This brittle bone disease puts vitamin D deficient individuals at a higher risk of getting bone fractures (Fleet, 2010). As you can see, vitamin D is an incredibly important nutrient we should all ensure we produce enough of.

Where Can I Find Vitamin D?

As we previously talked about, a major source of vitamin D is from our own bodies when we are exposed to direct sunlight. From late spring to early autumn, most of us will get all the vitamin D we need providing we spend enough time outdoors. It's not yet clear exactly how much time is necessary to spend out in the sun to produce an adequate amount of vitamin D. However, you will not have to spend your summer sunbathing if that is what you're wondering. Spending short periods of time in the sun regularly should allow your body to produce all the vitamin D it needs (NHS Choices, 2019).

While vitamin D can be produced in the body, it can also be found in a number of healthy foods. Seafood is a great source of vitamin D, with salmon, tuna, herring, and sardines being particularly nutritious options. Salmon and tuna are also rich in Omega-3 fatty acids which are known to have anticoagulant properties (ePainAssist, 2018). If you are not a fish lover, all is not lost, however. Vitamin D can also be found in abundance in egg yolks. Interestingly, the vitamin D content of an egg varies depending on how long the chicken that laid it spent in the sun! An alternative to seafood and egg yolks is vitamin supplements. A popular vitamin D supplement is cod liver oil. It is an excellent source of vitamin D and has been used for many years to treat vitamin D deficiencies in children (*7 Healthy Foods That Are High in Vitamin D*, 2019).

Chapter 5: Iron

It turns out that vitamins are not the only essential nutrients out there. You've also got minerals, and one of their biggest players is iron. Iron has important functions in the human body. Most notably, iron is an important component of hemoglobin, the substance in red blood cells that is responsible for ferrying oxygen from your lungs to the rest of your body. If you have an iron deficiency, your body cannot produce enough red blood cells to carry oxygen around your body. An iron deficiency can result in a person becoming increasingly fatigued. This iron deficiency-causing exhaustion can impact everything on your body, ranging from your immune system to your brain's ability to properly function (Watson, 2011).

Being an important component of the oxygen-carrying hemoglobin is not the only important function of iron; Iron is also important to the maintenance of healthy cells, skin, hair, and nails. Despite how important it is, an iron deficiency is quite common in comparison to other essential nutrients. It is the most common nutritional deficiency in the United States. According to the Centers for Disease Control and Prevention, roughly ten percent of women are not receiving their recommended 18mg of iron per day (Watson, 2011).

Chapter 6: Zinc

Yet another mineral that plays a vital role in the body's health is zinc. Unlike fat-soluble vitamins, the human body cannot produce nor store zinc. Instead, we must get a constant supply through our diet. This is important as zinc is essential to numerous bodily processes, including gene expression, protein production, wound healing, growth, enzymatic reactions, and the healing of wounds. Zinc is required for the activity of over 300 enzymes. These enzymes assist with metabolism, digestion, and the function of the nervous system (Kubala, 2018).

Additionally, zinc is important for the function of our taste and smell senses. Consequently, a zinc deficiency can result in a person's sense of taste or smell deteriorating, as one of the enzymes responsible for taste and smell depends on zinc. Symptoms of zinc deficiency include thinning hair, diarrhea, a poor immune system, a decreased appetite, mood disturbances, and impaired wound healing. It is estimated that approximately two billion people around the world are not getting enough zinc from their diet (Kubala, 2018).

Where Can I Find Iron and Zinc?

Now on to our two favorite minerals: Iron and zinc. Meat is an excellent source of both iron and zinc. Red meat is also a particularly good source, but high levels of iron and zinc can also be found in pork, beef, and lamb. Shellfish are also an excellent, low-calorie option high in iron and zinc. Oysters, crabs, mussels, and shrimp all contribute greatly to your daily iron and zinc intake. So, if you are a lover of shellfish and are watching your iron and zinc intake, you are in luck! Seeds are a surprisingly excellent source of iron and zinc; squash, pumpkin, and sesame seeds all have high zinc content and would make a fine addition to a balanced diet (*The 10 Best Foods That Are High in Zinc*, 2018). While fresh fruit is ordinarily an excellent go-to for vitamin intake, dried fruit is actually a superior option when it comes to iron. For example, dried apricots contain almost seven times more iron than fresh fruit! (*Top Foods High in Iron*, n.d.).

Conclusion

By now, you'll be well aware of the extent of the importance of vitamins and minerals. I hope this guide has been helpful and will assist you in making any potential change-ups to your diet, whether for the purposes of maximizing your vitamin and mineral intake or getting them from new and exciting foods. Learning about vitamins and minerals can be an interesting and fun exercise that reminds us just how extraordinary the human body is and how important it is to keep it that way.

References

B Vitamins. (2019, June 4). The Nutrition Source.

https://www.hsph.harvard.edu/nutritionsource/vitamins
/vitamin-b/

Brazier, Y. (2020, December 14). Vitamins: What are
they, and what do they do?

Www.medicalnewstoday.com.
https://www.medicalnewstoday.com/articles/195
878#soluble-in-fat-vs-water

Does garlic have vitamin B? (n.d.). Askinglot.com.
Retrieved July 28, 2021, from

https://askinglot.com/does-garlic-have-vitamin-b

ePainAssist, T. (2018, January 20). 14 Foods That Have
Anticoagulant Properties.

EPainAssist. https://www.epainassist.com/diet-and-
nutrition/foods-that-have-anticoagulant-
properties

Fleet, J. C. (2010, November 29). What is Vitamin D?
Www.youtube.com.

https://www.youtube.com/watch?v=zQcsoWTAxHo&t=5
    4s

Healthfully. (n.d.). Healthfully. Retrieved July 28, 2021,
    from

https://healthfully.com/339556-herbs-that-lower-blood-
    pressure-quickly.html

Kubala, J. (2018, November 14). Zinc: Everything You
    Need to Know. Healthline;

Healthline   Media.
    https://www.healthline.com/nutrition/zinc#defici
    ency

Mayo Clinic Staff. (2020, November 13). Vitamin A. Mayo
    Clinic;

https://www.mayoclinic.org/drugs-supplements-
    vitamin-a/art-20365945

M, K. (2008, April 8). The Benefits of Vitamin C.
    WebMD; WebMD.

https://www.webmd.com/diet/features/the-benefits-of-
    vitamin-c#1

National Institutes of Health. (2017). Office of Dietary Supplements - Vitamin A.

Nih.gov. https://ods.od.nih.gov/factsheets/VitaminA-HealthProfessional/

NHS Choices. (2019). How to get vitamin D from sunlight - Healthy body. NHS.

https://www.nhs.uk/live-well/healthy-body/how-to-get-vitamin-d-from-sunlight/

NHS Choices. (2019). Vitamin A - Vitamins and minerals. NHS.

https://www.nhs.uk/conditions/vitamins-and-minerals/vitamin-a/

Lehman, S. (2015, February 27). 15 Foods That Are High in Vitamin C. Verywell Fit;

Verywellfit. https://www.verywellfit.com/foods-high-in-vitamin-c-2507745

The 10 Best Foods That Are High in Zinc. (2018, April 19). Healthline.

https://www.healthline.com/nutrition/best-foods-high-in-zinc#TOC_TITLE_H

Top Foods High in Iron. (n.d.). WebMD. Retrieved July
28, 2021, from

https://www.webmd.com/diet/foods-high-in-iron#2

Vitamins & Minerals: What is Vitamin D? (n.d.).
Www.centrum.com. Retrieved July 27,

2021, from https://www.centrum.com/learn/vitamins-
minerals/vitamin-d/

Vitamin C: The Healing Power Of The Pineapple. (n.d.).
Www.streetdirectory.com.

Retrieved July 28, 2021, from
https://www.streetdirectory.com/food_editorials/
health_food/fruits/vitamin_c_the_healing_powe
r_of_the_pineapple.html#:~:text=Furthermore%
2C%20due%20to%20its%20high%20vitamin%20
C%20content%2C

Watson, S. (2011, July 13). What You Need to Know
About Iron Supplements. WebMD; WebMD.

https://www.webmd.com/vitamins-and-
supplements/features/iron-supplements

What does Vitamin B Do? | Foods & Sources | Holland &
     Barrett. (n.d.).

Www.hollandandbarrett.com.
     https://www.hollandandbarrett.com/the-health-
     hub/vitamins-and-
     supplements/vitamins/vitamin-b/what-does-
     vitamin-b-do/

What is vitamin C? (n.d.). BBC Good Food.

https://www.bbcgoodfood.com/howto/guide/what-
     vitamin-c

7 Healthy Foods That Are High in Vitamin D. (2019,
     December 19). Healthline.

https://www.healthline.com/nutrition/9-foods-high-in-
     vitamin-d#3.-Cod-liver-oil

15 Healthy Foods High in B Vitamins. (2018, October 11).
     Healthline.

https://www.healthline.com/nutrition/vitamin-b-
     foods#TOC_TITLE_HDR_3

Notes:

Notes:

Notes:

Notes:

www.ingramcontent.com/pod-product-compliance
Lightning Source LLC
Chambersburg PA
CBHW072346270726
48659CB00023B/2407